I0468486

Table of contents

Introduction

Women are a key partner for men and is involved with the development of society and the State and the world as a whole Renaissance factor in communities

To preserve the woman's health must be taken into account not only because they are in the labor market, but it liable for the stability of the family Mother is the first official teach children morals and love others, serve their communities and to promote their countries and help the poor and the lack of distinction between people of color or race, their learning also loves all people and this Requires attention to women's health , education from childhood on the meanings of goodness and beauty.Africa was one of the richest ancient continents, where a lot of wealth, but decades of colonialism, resulting in exhaustion, and depletion of these resources in several places in Africa and also factors is corruption, and pool Wealth in the hands of a few, spread ignorance, disease and civil war. Women in Africa are prey to ignorance, disease and exploitation during wars in this book collected most of the diseases affecting women in Africa that developed countries should assist these States, in particular the women that don't get simpler their food, health and work, respect.

Causes of poverty

1. Corruption,
2. Ethnic violence.
3. Free trade agreements against the African continent
4. Their lack of resources in the region.
5. Limited employment opportunities,
6. Poor infrastructure, poor roads, railways, water systems, etc., Yet these are some of the major drivers of economic development.
7. Poor resource usage.
8. Wars and unending conflicts, scaring the world investments.
9. Poor World Bank.
10. **POOR LAND UTILIZATION**. Educated on what to do with the land, because some people are just stuck in their rudimentary ways of doing things. Use the land to grow crops which are just enough for subsistence survival.Nothing goes to the market for sale.
11. **DISEASES AND POOR HEALTH FACILITIES**. Malaria, HIV/AIDS, TB. When the less resources are spent on treating the sick. In a worst case scenario where the breadwinner dies, those who are left behind have no resources to support themselves.
12. Many of the poorest nations in the world were former colonies, slave-exporting areas and territories from which

resources had been systematically extracted for the benefit of colonizing countries

13. **National Debt.** Many poor countries carry significant debt loads due to loans from wealthier nations and international financial institutions. Poorer nations pay an average of $2.30 in debt service for every $1 received in grant aid.

14. **Discrimination and social inequality.** Poverty and inequality are two different things, but inequality can feed widespread poverty by barring groups with lower social status from accessing the tools and resources to support themselves.

15. **Vulnerability to natural disasters.**

16. Traditional African healers have been using ritual and herbal remedies to treat people for centuries.

Women's health problems

- **Infectious disease**
- **Noninfectious diseases**
    1. **Malnutrition.**
    2. **War psychological problems**

Infectious diseases;

African women are exposed to many infectious diseases:

Risk Factors for infectious diseases:

Risk of AIDS

Transfusions, organ transplants, contaminated hypodermic apparatus, sexual transmission, vertical spread from infected mother to child

- Have unprotected sex
- Have multiple sex partners.
- Are a man who has sex with other men.
- Have high-risk partner(s) (partner has multiple sex partners, is a man who has sex with other men, or injects drugs).
- Have or have recently had a sexually transmitted disease, such as syphilis.

People, who inject drugs, or steroids, especially if they share needles, syringes, cookers, or other equipment used to inject drugs, are at risk of being infected with HIV.

Persons with Medical Conditions that Weaken the Immune System for TB

Babies and young children often have weak immune systems. Other people can have weak immune systems, too, especially people with any of these conditions:

- HIV infection (the virus that causes AIDS

- Substance abuse

- Silicosis

- Diabetes mellitus

- Severe kidney disease

- Low body weight

- Organ transplants

- Head and neck cancer

- Medical treatments such as corticosteroids or organ transplant

- Specialized treatment for rheumatoid arthritis or Crohn's disease

Risk factors for getting malaria include:

- Not taking medicine to prevent malaria Being outdoors, especially in rural areas, between dusk and dawn (nighttime), when the mosquitoes that transmit malaria are most active.
- In the absence of a vaccine of tropical diseases like malaria and with increasing travel from non-endemic to endemic countries malaria,

- Not taking steps for protection from mosquito bites.

  Your risk of getting malaria depends on your age, history of exposure to malaria, and whether you are pregnant. Most adults who have lived in areas where malaria is present have developed partial immunity to malaria because of previous infections and so almost never develop severe disease. But young children who live in these areas and travelers to these areas are especially at risk for malaria because they have not developed this immunity.

Risk of cholera

- **Poor sanitary conditions.** Cholera is more likely to flourish in situations where a sanitary environment — including a safe water supply — is difficult to maintain. Such conditions are common in refugee camps, impoverished countries, and areas devastated by famine, war or natural disasters.
- **Reduced or nonexistent stomach acid (hypochlorhydria or achlorhydria).** Cholera bacteria can't survive in an acidic environment, and ordinary stomach acid often serves as a first-

line defense against infection. But people with low levels of stomach acid — such as children, older adults, and people who take antacids, H-2 blockers or proton pump inhibitors — lack this protection, so they're at greater risk of cholera.

- **Household exposure.** There is increased risk of cholera with living with someone who has the disease.
- **Type O blood.** For reasons that aren't entirely clear, people with type O blood are twice as likely to develop cholera as are people with other blood types.
- **Raw or undercooked shellfish.** Although large-scale cholera outbreaks no longer occur in industrialized nations, eating shellfish from waters known to harbor the bacteria greatly increases your risk.
  - The lack of easy access to health clinics and the costs of certain treatments or prevention methods can put help out of the reach of many families.

Syphilis

- Engage in unprotected sex
- Have sex with multiple partners
- Are a man who has sex with men
- Are infected with HIV, the virus that causes AIDS

schistosomiasis

- *Schistosoma mansoni S. haematobium* distributed throughout Africa:

- There is a risk of infection in freshwater in southern and sub-Saharan Africa–including the great lakes and rivers as well as smaller bodies of water.

- Transmission also occurs in the Nile River valley in Egypt and the Mahgreb region of North Africa.

African trypanosomiasis

- Both forms of sleeping sickness are transmitted by the bite of the tsetse fly (*Glossina* species).
- Tsetse flies inhabit rural areas, living in the woodlands and thickets that dot the East African savannah. In central and West Africa, they live in the forests and vegetation along streams. Tsetse flies bite during daylight hours.
- Both male and female flies can transmit the infection, but even in areas where the disease is endemic, only a very small percentage of flies are infected.
- He vast majority of infections is transmitted by the tsetse fly, other modes of transmission are possible.
- A pregnant woman can pass the infection to her unborn baby
- The infection can also be transmitted by blood transfusion or sexual contact

Risk factors of polio

- The absence of immunization against the disease.
- Poor sanitation and sporadic or nonexistent immunization programs,
- Pregnant women.
- Very young.
- Weakened immune systems.
- Travel to an area where polio is common or that has recently experienced an outbreak
- Living with or caring for someone who may be shedding poliovirus
- A compromised immune system, such as occurs with HIV infection
- Having removed tonsils removed (tonsillectomy
- Extreme stress or strenuous physical activity after being exposed to poliovirus, both of which can depress your immune system.

Risk factors of Chagas disease

The following factors may increase the risk of getting Chagas disease:

- Living in impoverished rural areas of Central America, South America and Mexico
- Living in a residence that contains triatomine bugs.
- Receiving a blood transfusion or organ transplant from a person who carries the infection

Risk factors of Leishmania (Kala Azar)

Climate and other environmental changes have the potential to expand the geographic range of the sand fly vectors and the areas in the world where leishmaniasis is found.

Risk factors of leprosy

- People in constant physical contact with infected people.
- Genetic defects in the immune system may cause certain people to be more likely to become infected (region q25 on chromosome 6).
- Handling certain animals that are known to carry the bacteria (for example, armadillos, African chimpanzee, sooty mangabey, and cynomolgus

macaque) are at risk of getting the bacteria from the animals, especially if they do not wear gloves while handling the animals.

Risk of Exposure of Ebola

- Healthcare providers caring for Ebola patients and family and friends in close contact with Ebola patients are at the highest risk of getting sick because they may come in contact with infected blood or body fluids.

- Ebola also can be spread through direct contact with objects (like clothes, bedding, needles, syringes/sharps or medical equipment) that have been contaminated with infected body fluids. People can become sick with Ebola after coming in contact with infected wildlife.

- Ebola may spread as a result of handling bush meat (wild animals hunted for food) and contact with infected bats.

  Ebola could spread through sex or other contact with semen from men who have survived Ebola. Until more information is known, avoid contact with semen from a man who has had Ebola.

Sequels of infectious Diseases on women

Tuberculosis

- Tuberculosis is the single biggest infectious killer in women.
- TB is one of the top five killers of women among adult women aged 20–59 years. 480 000 women died from TB in 2014, including 140 000 deaths among women who were HIV-positive.
- It kills nearly 2 - 3 million people yearly.
- It is primarily a lung infection caused by inhalation of droplets containing tubercle bacilli of cough spray from tuberculosis patients.
- Mycobactarium tuberculosis and M. Arcanum are two predominant causative strains in Africa.
- In many Sub-Saharan African countries, especially Central and East Africa, the incidence of TB has increased with the advent and increasing occurrence of human immunodeficiency virus (HIV) seropositivity.
- In a number of these countries one in three people with HIV dies from TB due to neglect, they also infect hundreds of HIV-negative persons with TB bacteria.
- According to WHO Global Tuberculosis Program (GTP) recent reports over 900 million women are infected with TB world-wide and they are also at greater risk of HIV infection
- TB among mothers is associated with a sixfold increase in perinatal deaths and a twofold risk of premature birth and low birth-weight.
- Genital TB, which is challenging to diagnose, has been identified as an important cause of infertility in high TB-

incidence settings. TB in pregnant women living with HIV increases the

- Risk of maternal and infant mortality by almost 300%.
- In Africa, TB rates are up to 10 times higher in Pregnant women living with HIV than in pregnant women without HIV infection.
- Settings found TB accounted for 15-34% of the indirect causes of obstetric mortality. Evidence from India has found that TB among
- Mothers living with HIV, is associated with more than double the risk of vertical transmission of HIV to the unborn child.

Complications of TB on female genital tract

Pelvic TB

- Tuberculous adenitis, of either the mesenteric or the pelvic lymph nodes, without involvement of the genital tract.

- Generalized miliary peritoneal TB, in which grayish white tubercles stud the abdomen, may involve the serosal surface of both abdominal and pelvic organs without penetrating to the mucosa.

- Such superficial lesions do not usually impair the reproductive function of the pelvic organs.

Fallopian tubes TB

The Fallopian tubes constitute the initial focus of genital TB in the overwhelming majority of cases

In more than 90% of patients with genital TB, the tubes are involved bilaterally. Although only one tube appears infected, there probably are microscopic lesions in the other. In the early stages, the tubes show little change, but as progression occurs, the diameter of the tube becomes larger .

 The ampullary region shows the earliest and most extensive changes,

 the fimbrial processes become greatly swollen, and the ostia remain open or closed

Table 1. Frequency of tuberculosis in genital organs

Organ	Frequency (%)
Fallopian tubes	90–100
Endometrium	50–60

Organ	Frequency (%)
Ovaries	20–30
Cervix	5–15
Vulva and vagina	1

(From Schaefer, G: Female genital tuberculosis. Clin Obstet Gynecol 19:23, 1976)

TB of endometrium:

In genital TB, there is a high incidence of involvement of the endometrium

Grossly, the size and shape of the uterus may appear normal. The tuberculous process generally is localized to the endometrium, is most extensive in the fundus, and decreases toward the cervix.

- The myometrium is not usually involved.

- In premenopausal patients, much of the infected tissue is shed during the menstruation, only to have the endometrium reinfected from the tubes with each cycle.

- However, when extensive involvement of the endometrium occurs, there may be ulcerative, granular, or fungating lesions present, or the endometrial cavity may be obliterated with intrauterine adhesions

- Total destruction of the endometrium with resulting amenorrhea, secondary to end-organ failure and predisposition to pyometra should the internal OS become occluded.

TB of the ovary

Usually, the involvement is bilateral

Two forms of ovarian TB are described:

1. perioophoritis, in which the ovary may be surrounded by or encased in adhesions and studded with tubercles caused by direct extension from the tube.

2. oophoritis, in which infection starts in the stroma of the ovary, presumably from a hematogenous source that produces a caseating granuloma within the parenchyma.

Perioophoritis

- Extension of the tuberculous process from the tube involves the ovary in a tubo ovarian mass,

- Oophoritis is a relatively rare condition and usually follows hematogenous spread. Typical tubercles or larger foci with Cassius centers may be recognized in cross section in the hilum of the ovary.

TB of the cervix

- The cervix appears to be involved in 5–25% of cases, whereas involvement of the external genitalia occurs only rarely.

The most common type is the ulcerative form, although papillomatous and miliary forms may also occur.

Whereas ulceration or destruction of surface epithelium is less common.

Increased secretion of mucin.

TB of the vulva and vagina:

TB of the vulva and vagina is the rarest form of genital TB, occurring in less than 2% of cases

In the vulva, it begins as a nodule on the labia or in the vestibular region, which breaks down and forms an irregular ragged ulcer, sometimes with sinuses discharging caseous material and pus.

TB of Bartholin's gland is rare.

A vulvar lesion presents as a hypertrophic, irregular warty growth sometimes resembling elephantiasis.

A tuberculous lesion in the vagina may simulate carcinoma in its gross appearance.

Tuberculous peritonitis:

Extensive adhesions are seen in patients with pelvic TB.

Two types of tuberculous peritonitis have been described:

1. The plastic variety, and is characterized by tender abdominal masses and an abdomen "doughy" to palpation.

2. The serous variety. The serous variety is seen more commonly and is characterized by ascitis, signs of peritoneal inflammation, fever, abdominal pain, weight loss, and anorexia. Chills, fever, ascitis, and sometimes, rebound tenderness. In the plastic variety, one may observe symptoms suggestive of partial intestinal obstruction.

Clinical features

- Tuberculous pleurisy, peritonitis, erythema nodosum, or renal, osseous, or pulmonary TB.

- A history of poor general health persisting over months or years and associated with weight loss, undue fatigue, low-grade fever, or vague lower abdominal discomfort is often elicited in patients with genital TB.

- Female genital TB is typically understood as a disease of young women, with 80% to 90% of cases diagnosed in patients 20–40 years old, often during work-up for subfertility.

- Although in many developing countries, genital TB is more common among younger women, in developed countries most patients are older than 40 years.

Table 2. Symptoms related to genital tuberculosis

Systemic

    Weight loss
    Fatigue
    Low-grade fever

Infertility

    Primary, Secondary

Menstrual disturbances

    Amenorrhea
    Menorrhagia

Metrorrhagia

Oligomenorrhea

Abdominal swelling

Postcoital bleeding

Vaginal discharge

Dyspareunia

Menstrual Disorders

- Abnormal uterine bleeding in genital TB has been reported in 10% to 40% of patients. Patients report menorrhagia, menometrorrhagia, intermenstrual bleeding, oligomenorrhea, and postmenopausal bleeding.

- Other symptoms seen less frequently with pelvic TB include vaginal discharge, abdominal swelling, pelvic relaxation, and symptoms associated with fistula formation.

- Uterovesical, tubointestinal, and tuboperitoneal fistulas have all been described.

- TB is significant because it may affect any organ in the body, may exist without manifesting clinical signs and symptoms, and may recur after being apparently arrested.

- Genital TB can mimic ovarian cancer.

- These patients commonly present with adnexal masses and ascitis.

Physical signs in genital tuberculosis

- Normal

- Abdominal mass

- Pelvic Mass

- Adnexal mass

- Abdominal tenderness

- Pelvic/adnexal tenderness

- Ascites

- Excessive vaginal discharge

- Ulcer in the vulva, vagina, and cervix

- Enlarged uterus with pyometra
  Fistula

Complication of genital TB in women

Subfertility or Sterility

Extensive damage to the Fallopian tubes and the endometrium is often irreversible, and chances of successful intrauterine pregnancy drop significantly. TB today.

Ectopic Pregnancy

The damage to the Fallopian tubes can be extensive and irreparable if genital TB is not diagnosed and treated early in its course. After medical treatment, the risk of ectopic pregnancy in patients with pelvic TB is estimated to be 33–72%.

Congenital Tuberculosis

- Serious complication of female genital TB is congenital TB. Maternal tuberculous endometrium to the fetus are rare,

- Congenital TB can be an overwhelming systemic infection in the newborn and has considerable morbidity and mortality if untreated.

Perinatal outcome of pregnancy following treatment for genital tuberculosis

- The prevalence of TB, especially extrapulmonary TB, is increasing worldwide. However, we know little about the outcome of pregnancy.

- Tuberculous adenitis did not affect the course of pregnancy or labor or the perinatal outcome compared with the control group: 21 women with other extrapulmonary lesions had higher rates of antenatal hospitalization (24% versus 2%) and infants with low Apgar scores (less than or equal to 6) and low-birth-weight (less than 2500 g) infants (33% versus 11%).

- Extrapulmonary TB lesions other than lymph adenitis are associated with adverse outcome following pregnancy and childbirth.

Malaria

- <u>Malaria</u> is widespread and kills one African child every 30 seconds. It is the leading cause of death among under-fives in many countries.
- Malaria is caused by parasites that are transmitted to people through the bites of infected female mosquitoes. *P. falciparum.*
- It is the most deadly malaria parasite and the most prevalent in Africa,
- The first symptoms of malaria usually appear between 10
- Fever, headache, chills and vomiting –and 15 days after the mosquito bite
- Severe illness and death.

Malaria in pregnant women

- Malaria infection during pregnancy is a significant public health problem
- Malaria is the result of *Plasmodium falciparum* infection and occurs predominantly in Africa.
- The risks are for the pregnant woman, her fetus, and the newborn child.
- Malaria-associated maternal illness
- Low birth weight.

Factors control the symptoms and complications of malaria in pregnancy:

1. Intensity in the given geographical area.
2. The individual's level of acquired immunity.

There are two transmission setting:

1. High-transmission settings

- In high-transmission settings, where levels of acquired immunity tend to be high, *P. falciparum* infection is usually asymptomatic in pregnancy.
- The adverse effects of *P. falciparum* infection in pregnancy is most pronounced for women in their first pregnancy.
- Parasites may be present in the placenta and contribute to maternal anemia even in the absence of documented peripheral parasitemia.
- Both maternal anemia and placental parasitemia can lead to low birth weight, which is an important contributor to infant mortality

Low-transmission settings

- Women of reproductive age have relatively little acquired immunity to malaria

- Malaria in pregnancy is associated with anemia
- An increased risk of severe malaria,
- Spontaneous abortion
- Stillbirth
- Prematurity and low birth weight.
- Malaria affects all pregnant women, regardless of the number of times they have been pregnant.

Infections with P. vivax

- Infection with *P. vivax*, as with *P. falciparum*, leads to chronic anemia and placental malaria infection, reducing the birth weight and increasing the risk of neonatal death.
- Women in their first pregnancy, the reduction in birth weight is approximately two thirds of what is associated with *P. falciparum*, but with *P. Viva* the effect appears to increase with successive pregnancies

Hepatitis B

Hepatitis B is a serious disease that attacks the liver.
Signs and symptoms include jaundice, fatigue, abdominal pain, loss of appetite, nausea, vomiting, and joint pain. Long-term complications of hepatitis B can include lifelong infection, scarring of the liver, liver cancer, liver failure, and death.
Hepatitis B is transmitted through sexual contact, sharing needles, and from mother to baby during childbirth.

Ninety percent of infants who are infected at birth will develop chronic hepatitis B infection.

15% to 20% will die from liver disease.

Hepatitis C virus HCV:

- Africa has the highest WHO estimated regional HCV prevalence (5.3%). Egypt has the highest prevalence (17.5%) of HCV in the world. Genotypes commonly found in Africa are 1, 4 and 5. Genotype 3 is found in Egypt and parts of Central Africa.

- Hepatitis C virus (HCV) is an RNA virus known to infect humans and chimpanzees, causing similar disease in these 2 species. HCV is most often transmitted parenterally, but is also transmitted vertically and sexually . HCV is up to 4 times more infectious than Human Immunodeficiency Virus (HIV). It also requires less exposure that HIV to cause infection .

- HCV is a leading cause of chronic liver disease in the world.

Pregnancy and hepatitis c:

- Pregnancy will not affect the course of the hepatitis, unless a woman has hepatitis E, which can worsen severely in some cases.

- Pregnancy itself **will not** accelerate the disease process .

- The liver is already burdened, and scarred with cirrhosis.

- The extra demands of pregnancy may predispose the expectant mother to a condition called acute fatty liver of pregnancy.

1. **Acute fatty liver of pregnancy**

- Acute fatty liver of pregnancy may be related to liver disease, deficiency of an enzyme normally produced by the liver that allows the pregnant woman to metabolize fatty acid.

- This condition can quickly become severe, and also affect the unborn child (who may also be born with a deficiency in this enzyme).

- The treatment is a quick delivery, and treatment in intensive care.

- Normally, the pregnant woman will recover quickly after the birth, and has a good prognosis if the liver damage is not severe.

2. **Cholelithiasis**:

It creates jaundice during pregnancy. It occurs in 6 % of so the risk of gallstones goes up.

Polio:

- Polio, now eradicated from many parts of the world, is still endemic in Nigeria and outbreaks also occur in other African countries.
- **Polio** or **infantile paralysis**, is an infectious disease caused by the poliovirus.
- In about 0.5% of cases there is muscle weakness resulting in an inability to move.
- This can occur over a few hours to a few days.
- The weakness most often involves the legs, but may less commonly involve the muscles of the head, neck and diaphragm. Many but not all people fully recover.
- In those with muscle weakness about 2% to 5% of children and 15% to 30% of adults die. Once contracted, it is incurable and can cause permanent paralysis.

Polio and pregnancy

- Most poliovirus infections are mild. However, pregnant women have been shown to be more susceptible to polio, with a higher chance of dying from the disease.

- Poliovirus affects the central nervous system, and can range from mild symptoms like headaches to severe symptoms like paralysis.

Elephantiasis,

Elephantiasis, which causes an accumulation of fluid, usually in a limb,

Leprosy

- Leprosy, which causes disfiguring skin sores and nerve damage

- High levels of steroids, thyroid hormones, and estrogen during pregnancy decrease cellular immunity, which reverses around the 12th week after childbirth.
- The period of immunosuppression between the last trimester of pregnancy and the first 3 months after childbirth increases predisposition to infection with *Mycobacterium leprae*and the reactivation of *M.*
- *leprae* in women who were apparently cured[1]. Complications in children born to women with leprosy include lower birth weight, smaller placenta, slow growth, increased incidence of infection, and mortality in childhood.

Pregnant women and leprosy :

- anemia and uterine height, because the antibacterial drug dapsone, used in the treatment of leprosy, can cause hemolytic anemia. This, together with the physiological anemia that develops during pregnancy, can have serious direct consequences for the mother and indirect consequences for the child, because it decreases the blood supply necessary for proper placental development
- Newborn with low birth weight.
- Emergence of leprosy reaction.
- Aggravation of leprosy toward the lepromatous pole.
- Relapse.
- Increased childhood infections.
- Other (aggravation of leprosy reaction, exfoliative dermatitis in the infant, premature newborn.

Helminthiasis

Helminthiasis, an infestation of parasitic worms in the intestines.

Factors of high incidence of helminthiasis

1) Insufficient public health education,
2) Poor personal and food hygiene,
3) Nonadherence to the rules of cattle-farming and keeping pets, and others.
4) In the majority of cases, people are found unaware of risks and complications of helminthiasis, and means of prevention against helminthic infestation.

Helminthiases are difficult to identify since they are often manifested by nonspecific

Signs of Helminthiases:

- Acne-form rash on the face.
- Stomach aches.
- Pains in the epigastrium.
- evacuatory disorders (constipation or diarrhea),
- Chronic fatigue syndrome.
- Joint aches.
- Dizziness.

Severe complications:

- Obturation of bile duct.
- The abscesses of liver and pancreas.
- Intestinal obstruction.
- Appendicitis.
- Rupture of the intestines.
- Affections of the central nervous system.
- Anemia.

Gynecological disorders

- Unusual appearance, amount, and smell of vaginal discharge,
- Discomforts in the region of external genitalia (burning sensations, itching) which affect the well-being and sexual intercourse in female patients.
- Presence of helmets and their eggs is an etiological factor of colitis.

- Relapsing copyrights' and latent infections (chlamydiosis, mycoplasmosis, and ureaplasmosis

- During pregnancy, through adverse effects on maternal anemia and on birth outcomes,
- Anti helminthic treatment during pregnancy will therefore be particularly beneficial

Trachoma

Trachoma is a bacterial eye infection which can lead to blindness.

If neglected, most diseases will cause severe debilitation which limits the sufferer's ability to earn a living. Early diagnosis and cures are available, but diseases continue to disable and claim the lives of many.

Diseases have a high acute mortality rate among women

a. Meningitis
b. Tetanus
c. Diarrhea
d. Mumps
e. Measles
f. Malaria
g. Lower respiratory infection

Chronic infections increase women's mortality:

a. Rheumatic heart disease.

b. Cancer cervix.

Risk factors increase the incidence of woman's exposure

1. Malnutrition

2. AIDS.

3. TB

4. Pregnancy.

5. Asthma

6. Rheumatic heart disease

7. Liver and kidney diseases.

8. Lack of vaccinations.

9. Lack of antenatal care.

10. Lack of early treatment.

Meningitis

- **Meningitis** is an <u>acute</u> <u>inflammation</u> of the protective membranes covering the brain and spinal cord.

- The inflammation may be caused by infection with <u>viruses</u>, <u>bacteria</u>

- Meningococcal disease can refer to any illness that is caused by the type of bacteria called Neisseria meningitides.

- Meningococcus bacteria are spread through the exchange of respiratory and throat secretions like spit (e.g., By living in close quarters, kissing). Meningococcal disease can be treated with antibiotics.

Chronic meningitis, especially with AIDS patients:

- o Tuberculous
- o Cryptococcal
- o Syphilitic
- o *Listeria* species
- o Lymphomatous
- o Aseptic

<u>Symptoms are:</u>

- Fever, headache and neck stiffness.

- Confusion or altered consciousness, vomiting,

- An inability to tolerate light or loud noises.

- Irritability, drowsiness, or poor feeding.

- Meningococcal bacteria a rash is present.

Meningitis complications are:

Deafness,

Epilepsy,

Hydrocephalus

Cognitive deficits

.

Diarrhea disease

o HIV infection has added considerably to the burden of diarrheal diseases among women

o This is of particular importance in African countries that show high HIV prevalence.

o It is difficult to quantify comorbidity and its contribution to the mortality.

o Because of the probable influence of HIV/AIDS, especially in the mortality due to diarrheal disease,

WHO divides of the African region into two subregions, according to mortality levels

- AFR D sub region (high child and high adult mortality)

- AFR E sub region (high child and very high adult mortality). Stratum E includes the countries in Sub-Saharan Africa, where HIV/AIDS has had a substantial impact.

Tetanus

- Maternal and neonatal tetanus (MNT) is a devastating disease caused by toxins released from Clostridium tetani bacteria.
- MNT is responsible for an average 110,000 deaths a year in the African Region.
- Once contracted, the newborn usually dies within seven days.

- However, MNT is entirely preventable through appropriate immunization of women of childbearing age, and through simple and basic precautionary measures in child delivery.

- Transmission occurs when there is contact between the bacteria and broken skin or dead tissues, such as the wound resulting when an infant's umbilical cord is cut.
- Poor hygienic conditions, lack of access to sterilized childbirth delivery tools, unhygienic practices, and limited

access to health services amplify the risk for MNT during childbirth.

Measles, mumps, and rubella:

o Measles, mumps, and rubella are viral diseases that may adversely affect non-immune pregnant women and their fetuses/neonates.

o Measles-mumps-rubella (MMR) vaccination before to pregnancy Prevent these diseases and their complications.

o The vaccine is contraindicated during pregnancy because it contains live, attenuated viruses that pose a risk to the fetus.

o Accidental receipt of MMR vaccination is not known to cause maternal/fetal complications.

o MMR immunization is recommended for non-immune obstetric patients upon completion or termination of pregnancy

Complications of Measles:

o Measles-induced complications affect approximately 30% of infected individuals, adults (Ages $\geq$ 20).

o The most commonly reported complications are diarrhea (8%), otitis media (7%), and pneumonia (6%).

o The leading cause of death in adults is acute encephalitis, a rare complication of measles (0.1%).

- Data suggest that complications are more severe in pregnant women.
- Measles exposure during pregnancy may cause adverse maternal and fetal effects.
- If a non-immune pregnant patient is exposed to measles just before delivery, in utero and intrapartum viral transmission is likely to cause a serious infection in the neonate.
- The risk can be reduced by passive immunization.

Mumps:

- Mumps, like measles, is a disease caused by an RNA virus classified in the *Paramyxoviridae* family.

- Mumps belong to the Rubulavirus genus

Complications in the obstetric patient

- If exposure occurs during the first trimester, the patient has a higher risk of spontaneous abortion.

- Spontaneous abortion has been found to occur in 27% of pregnant women exposed to mumps during their first trimester compared to 13% of controls.

- There are no associated congenital malformations in children whose mothers were exposed to mumps at any time during pregnancy.

Rubella

Rubella, or German measles, is an RNA virus in the genus Rubivirus within the *Togaviridae* family.

It is a human disease with no animal reservoirs.

Complications in the obstetric patient:

- Acquired rubella infection is generally mild.

- Transplacental passage of the virus to the embryo/fetus during maternal viremia (five to seven days after exposure) can cause a shocking penalty (i.e., CRS).

- Virus transmission with maternal re-infections is rare.

Chronic rubella syndrome (CRS):

CRS symptoms include:

- o Fetal death,

- o Spontaneous abortion.

- o Premature delivery

- o Ocular abnormalities (e.g., Cataracts and microophthalmia)

- o Neurological problems (e.g., Intellectual disability)

- o Abnormal cardiac development a

- o Most commonly, deafness. Congenital malformations may be present at birth or sometimes develop months to years after birth.

Delayed CRS-induced maladies are:

1. Type I diabetes mellitus

2. Deafness

3. Intellectual disability,

   Sub acute encephalitis.

4. The frequency and severity of CRS decrease as gestation progresses.

5. Maternal exposure to rubella during the first 12 weeks of pregnancy results in CRS in 85% of developing embryos/fetuses.

6. After 20th gestational week, the risk of congenital defects is minimal.

7. Neonatal rubella infections are possible when non-immune mothers transmit rubella to the fetus close to delivery.

AIDS

- HIV/AIDS infection in South Africa is distinctly divided along racial lines: 13.6% of black Africans in South Africa are HIV-positive, whereas only 0.3% of whites living in South Africa have the disease. [9] False traditional beliefs about HIV/AIDS,

- HIV/AIDS is more prevalent among female adults under the age of 40 in nearly all age groups. Roughly 4 in every 5 people with HIV/AIDS aged 20–24 are women, and only one third of people with HIV/AIDS aged 25–29 are men.

- Although prevalence is higher among women in general, only 1 in every 6 HIV/AIDS infected people with multiple sex partners are women.

- HIV prevalence among pregnant women is highest in the populous

- The latest HIV data collected at antenatal clinics suggest that HIV infection levels might be levelling off, with HIV prevalence in pregnant women at 30% in 2007, 29% in 2006, and 28% in 2007.

- The decrease in the percentage of young pregnant women (15–24 years) found to be infected with HIV also suggests a possible decline in the annual number of new infections

CENTRAL NERVOUS SYSTEM COMPLICATIONS

- Advanced HIV infection can lead to opportunistic infections of the brain and spinal cord . Well-known pathogens include *Toxoplasma gondii.* Cryptococcus neoformans, and JC virus.

- Primary central nervous system lymphoma may also affect severely immunocompromised patients.

- Infections and malignancy cause variable neurologic symptoms, usually reflecting the location and severity of disease

- Patients with solitary lesions often present with headache or focal deficits,

- Patients with increased intracranial pressure from substantial masses (with or without edema) may have visual disturbances, nausea, or altered consciousness.

- Patients with meningitis or encephalitis generally present with one or more of the following: fever, headache, neck pain or stiffness, altered mental status, or seizure.

- Symptoms of myelopathy include weakness and sensory changes; upper motor neuron signs, such as spasticity and hyperreflexia.

Cardiopulmonary System

CARDIOVASCULAR COMPLICATIONS

- Higher rates of myocardial infarction and atherosclerosis in patients with HIV infection.

- HIV appears to independently increase the risk of cardiovascular disease via elevated cytokine levels, chronic vascular inflammation, and endothelial dysfunction.

- Other cardiac complications (i.e., Cardiomyopathy, myocarditis, and pericarditis) are still reported, although their incidence has decreased as combination antiretroviral therapy has become widespread.

- Infective endocarditis occurs almost exclusively in those who use injection drugs.

PULMONARY COMPLICATIONS

- *Pneumocystis jiroveci* (formerly *Pneumocystis carinii*) pneumonia

- Patients with *P. jiroveci* pneumonia classically present with fever, progressive exertional dyspnea, and nonproductive cough.

- Rates of pulmonary arterial hypertension, chronic obstructive pulmonary disease, and lung cancer have remained the same or increased in patients with HIV infection over the past few decades. Exertional dyspnea, fatigue, cough, edema are the main symptoms.

- The effect of combination antiretroviral therapy on the clinical course and prognosis of HIV-associated pulmonary hypertension remains uncertain.

- HIV accelerates emphysema-associated processes in patients who smoke, leading to earlier development and high rates of chronic obstructive pulmonary disease.

- HIV also appears to raise the risk of lung cancer, even independent of smoking

Gastrointestinal and Hepatic Systems

- Candidal infection often affects the oral cavity, leading to dysphagia or odynophagia or the esophagus, manifesting as sharp or burning substernal discomfort.

- Aphthous ulcers and oral ulcers/esophagitis caused by cytomegalovirus or herpes simplex virus may also occur

- oropharyngeal cancer, given the prevalence of oral human papillomavirus

- Diarrhea is a common symptom in adults with HIV infection.

- Slightly higher rates of inflammatory bowel disease have been reported in patients with HIV infection.

PANCREATIC AND HEPATOBILIARY COMPLICATIONS

- HIV-associated pancreatitis is now primarily caused by antiretroviral use and hypertriglyceridemia, rather than opportunistic infections.

- Although acalculous cholecystitis may occur, the incidence of cholelithiasis does not appear to be increased by HIV.

- Chronic liver disease from viral or nonviral hepatitis has become a leading cause of morbidity and mortality in patients with HIV infection; patients should be screened for viral hepatitis at the time of HIV diagnosis.

- Nonalcoholic fatty liver disease is associated with various factors, including visceral adiposity, insulin resistance, dyslipidemia, and mitochondrial toxicity.

- Hepatocellular carcinoma.

Genital infection

- Genital herpes increases the risk of HIV transmission; studies have yet to confirm whether suppressive herpes treatment reduces this risk.

- Elevated rates of high-risk human papillomavirus subtypes are found in patients with HIV infection, increasing their risk of anogenital tract dysplasia.

Renal complications

- Acute and subacute complications related to antiretroviral therapy, such as a protease inhibitor–associated nephrolithiasis and nephrotoxicity from tenofovir (Viread) use, continue to occur.

- Rates of end-stage kidney disease caused by HIV-associated nephropathy has stabilized

- Diabetes, hypertension, and hepatitis C are emerging as major risk factors for chronic kidney disease in patients with HIV infection.

Metabolic and Endocrine Complications

- Glucose metabolism, lipid metabolism, adipose tissue distribution is insulin resistance, diabetes, dyslipidemia, and lipodystrophy can occasionally be attributed to antiretroviral therapy.

- These complications reflect complex interactions between the patient and traditional risk factors, medication effects, and infection (HIV causes chronic inflammation, immune system activation.

- Disorders of the hypothalamic-pituitary-adrenal and gonadal axes have been reported in patients with HIV infection.

- Central nervous system lesions can involve the hypothalamus and pituitary gland, leading to adrenal insufficiency and hypogonadism.

- Adrenal insufficiency is usually mild and may also be caused by direct HIV infection of the adrenals, disseminated opportunistic infections, malignancy, or medication use (e.g., Systemic ketoconazole [Nizoral]).

- Women with HIV infection commonly experience irregular menses and may be at higher risk of amenorrhea or premature ovarian failure.

Musculoskeletal System

- A three- to sixfold increased risk of reduced bone mineral density in patients with HIV infection.

- Various antiretrovirals have been associated with osteopenia and osteoporosis.

- o Other factors (e.g., Weight, nadir CD4 lymphocyte count, menopausal status, chronic steroid use) may play a role.

- o Patients with HIV infection are also vulnerable to osteomalacia and osteonecrosis, the latter involving ischemic subchondral bone tissue death.

- o Osteonecrosis typically manifests as joint pain or stiffness, particularly in the groin, hips, or shoulders

- o Extensive avascular necrosis with flattening of the right femoral head in a patient with osteonecrosis of the hips.

- o Myopathy from older nucleoside analogues may now be less common because of the availability of newer agents.

- o HIV also causes an autoimmune-mediated myopathy.

Lowe respiratory infection:

- Acute respiratory infections (ARI), particularly lower respiratory tract infections (LRTI
- The causative organism is bacteria, such as *Haemophilus influenza* type b (Hib) and *Streptococcus* Forty-two percent of these ARI-associated deaths occur in Africa.
- The HIV epidemic in many countries of Sub-Saharan.

Risk factors associated with increased susceptibility to LRTI women:

o Adequate housing, electricity

o Running tap water.

o Exposure to such risk factors as indoor smoke pollution

o Overcrowding in households

Lower respiratory infection causes deaths by 38% in African female while it is 27% in male.

There are 3 causes of lower respiratory infections:

Bacterial

Viral

Environmental

o Indoor cooking, which creates giant clouds of smoke from the traditional three stone wood fires and charcoal.

o Lanterns being used for light at night using kerosene

o The smoke wears down the lining of the lungs make it susceptible to disease and kills the cilia, which are in the upper respiratory tract.

o As the smoke causes paralysis of the cilia the pollutants enter the lungs without anything to stop it.

o   As women and children are in the smoke of the kitchen more than the men if affects them most severely. This explains the high rate of morbidity and mortality due to lung diseases.

Very minors are these diseases caused by smoking cigarettes in Africa.

African women's mortality due to chronic infection

I.   Rheumatic heart disease

Predisposing factors are poverty, malnutrition, overcrowding, poor housing and a shortage of health care resources

o   Rheumatic heart disease is cardiac inflammation and scarring triggered by an autoimmune reaction to infection with group A streptococci.

Acute stage, this condition consists of pancarditis, involving inflammation of the myocardium, endocardium, and epicardium.

Chronic disease is manifested by valvular fibrosis, resulting in stenosis and/or insufficiency.

<u>Rheumatic fever</u> :

o   Acute rheumatic fever (ARF) and rheumatic heart disease (RHD) remain major causes of heart failure, stroke and death among African women and children, despite being preventable and eminently treatable.

o   From 21 to 22 February 2015, the Social Cluster of the Africa Union Commission (AUC) hosted a consultation with RHD experts convened by the Pan-African Society of Cardiology (PASCAR) in Addis Ababa, Ethiopia, to develop a 'roadmap' of key actions that need to be taken by governments to eliminate ARF and eradicate RHD in Africa.

o   It is rare before age 5 years and after age 25 years; it is most frequently observed in children and adolescents.

o   Rheumatic heart disease (RHD) remains a major public health problem in developing countries.

o   Half of the 2.4 million children affected by RHD globally live on the Africa.

o   RHD accounts for a major proportion of all cardiovascular disease in

o   Children and young adults in African countries.

- While acute rheumatic fever is on the decline even in the developing world, there are still a large number of chronic rheumatic heart disease cases in

- Africa complicated by chronic congestive heart failure and recurrent thrombo-embolic phenomena, both posing greater challenges for management.

- Pregnant women with rheumatic heart disease of moderate-severe mitral stenosis, severe pulmonary hypertension and atrial fibrillation are at high risk of heart failure.

Cardiac complications of rheumatic heart disease

1. Functional TR

2. Pulmonary hypertension

3. Left ventricular thrombus

4. Valvular cardiomyopathy
5. Infective endocarditis
6. Atrial fibrillation
7. Chronic congestive heart failure and recurrent thrombo-embolic phenomena, both posing greater challenges for management.

Pregnancy with rheumatic heart diseases

Pregnant women with rheumatic heart disease of moderate-severe mitral stenosis, severe pulmonary hypertension and atrial fibrillation are at high risk of heart failure.

- The fetal outcome is not good class III and IV. Heart disease is a leading cause of maternal death worldwide. Western countries

- In developing countries, rheumatic heart disease and its long-term consequences are more important..

Cancer cervix

- Infection of the cervix with human papillomavirus (HPV) is the most common cause of cervical cancer. However, not all women with an HPV infection will develop cervical cancer.

- Human papilloma virus (HPV) is the major cause of the main types of cervical cancer – squamous cell cancer and adenocarcinoma.

- There are over 100 different types of human papilloma virus (HPV). At least 40 types are passed on through sexual contact. Some types are called the wart virus or genital wart virus because they cause genital warts. The types of HPV that cause warts do not usually cause cell changes that develop into cancer.

- At least 15 types of HPV are considered high risk for cancer of the cervix - they include types 16 and 18. These 2 types cause about 7 out of 10 cancers of the cervix (70%).

- **Risk factors for cancer cervix:**

1. Persistent infections with high risk types of HPV.

2. Many sexual partners. The greater the number of sexual partners — and the greater the partner's number of sexual partners — the greater your chance of acquiring HPV.

3. Early sexual activity.

4. Other sexually transmitted infections (STIs). ...

5. A weak immune system

a. AIDS

b. TB

c. Immunosuppressive drugs.

d. Emotional stress.

e. Physical stressors.

f. Environmental and occupational chemical exposure.

g. UV and other types of radiation.

h. Common viral or bacterial infections.

i. Malnutrition has an impact on immune response.

j. Inadequate protein, calorie, vitamin, mineral

k. Water intake fosters decreased immune performance as well.

l. The biological state of aging counteracts immune function, particularly after age of 40

6. Smoking

7. Women who have had three or more full-term pregnancies, or who had their first full-term pregnancy before age 17, are twice as likely to get cervical cancer.

8. Women with a sister or mother who had cervical cancer are two to three times more likely to develop cervical cancer.

9. Women who take oral contraceptives for more than five years have an increased risk of cervical cancer, but this risk returns to normal within a few years after the pills are stopped.

10. Women who take oral contraceptives for more than five years have an increased risk of cervical cancer, but this risk returns to normal within a few years after the pills are stopped.

11. Genetic factor

- Women All cancer has a genetic basis since it is triggered by mutations (changes) in the genes of a cell.

- Genetic changes can have many causes. Most cancers occur by sporadically. For instance, gene changes may result from a random mistake when cells are dividing.

- Genes may also change in response to lifestyle habits (e.g., diet, exercise) and/or environment exposures or injuries.

- A small portion—about five to 10 percent—of cancers have been identified as resulting from genetic changes that are inherited. Inherited cancers occur when the cancer-causing gene alterations are passed from parent to child.

.

Women and civil war:

Economic effects of civil war

It increases poverty by

1. **Agriculture**

- **Spoiling farmland**

- **The farmers are busy with the war and the death of many of them**

- Lack of agricultural equipment agricultural machinery pills
  The lack of roads and safe corridors for transportation of crops.

2. Industry

- Stop factories lack the machinery and accessories industry

- Destroy factories during the war.

1. Trade
Stop importing and export with States for lack of means of land, sea and air.

2. Social sequel of civil war on women

- The loss of husband and breadwinner in the war leading to the impoverishment of the family.

- Women exposed to severe psychological pressure as a result of the loss of sons and brothers and scattered family.

3. **Medical sequel of civil war on women**

   - Women exposed to poverty and neglect.

   - Famine and food shortages.

   - Disability and lost legs or grow as a result of the war.

   - The spread of diseases and the absence of vaccinations.

   - Rape, and AIDS transmission.

   - The lack of health care during pregnancy and childbirth .
     Fetal abortion.

   - Bleeding, infection after childbirth
     Intrauterine fetal death ,and preeclampsia

How to help African women

General recommendations:

- Stop the wars and reconciliation

- Overall development

- All global institutions take their ethical responsibility and assist the development of these countries.

- Awareness and education for women and girls.

- Provide food and clean water.

- Provision of sewerage and sanitation infrastructure for receiving.

- Provide healthy homes

- Providing medical care for pregnant women and provide vaccinations crisis

- Efficient services and special effort by health providers is needed to enhance the health status of populations in this region.

- Planning for health services, improving the efficiency and engendering services in any country depends primarily on information about the main causes of ill-health and death in defined areas.

- Data on cause-specific mortality and morbidity, in particular, data disaggregated by gender and sex crucial for effective planning are scanty for most countries in sub-Saharan Africa (Heggengougen 1996).

- Gaining solid and longitudinal understanding across the life span based on reliable, consistent and quality data has been re-echoed as perhaps the first action for tackling major causes of ill-health (Stephens 1996).

- Given the paucity of data available to health planners in Africa.

Specific measures according to specific diseases

Measures for AIDS and TB

- Remove underlying risk factors and assure gender-equitable access

- Services for TB prevention, diagnosis, treatment, care and support.
- TB, HIV, maternal, neonatal and child health programs and primary care services should collaborate to maximize for women at all levels.
- Integrate TB screening and (investigation into reproductive health services, including family planning, antenatal and postnatal care.
- Care be given to girls and women living with HIV in high HIV and TB prevalent settings.
- Improve the recording and (reporting of TB data disaggregated by sex and age.
- Monitoring systems for HIV, PMTCT and TB care to capture data and ensure successful follow-up of the patient with HIV and TB prevalent settings.
- TB diagnosis in people living with HIV or who are suspected of multidrug- resistant TB.
- Increased research for the development of new diagnostics and new drugs which also take into account the specific needs of women living with HIV as well as pregnant and lactating women, as well as relevant operational and social science research.

WHO recommends the following package of interventions for the prevention and treatment of malaria during pregnancy:

- Use of long-lasting insecticidal nets (LLINs);

- In areas of stable malaria transmission of sub-Saharan Africa, intermittent preventive treatment in pregnancy (IPTp) with sulfadoxine-pyrimethamine (SP);
- Prompt diagnosis and effective treatment of malaria infections.

Intermittent preventive treatment in pregnancy

- Routine antenatal care.
- IPTp reduces maternal malaria episodes, maternal anemia, placental parasitemia, low birth weight, and neonatal mortality.
- All pregnant women should receive iron and folic acid supplementation.

Measures for Meningitis

- Some forms of meningitis are preventable by immunization with the meningococcal, mumps, pneumococcal, and Hib vaccines.
- Giving antibiotics to people with significant exposure to certain types of meningitis may also be useful.
- The first treatment of acute meningitis consists of promptly giving antibiotics and sometimes antiviral drugs.
- Corticosteroids can also be used to prevent complications from excessive inflammation.

Measures for prevention of lower respiratory infections

- The best way to prevent this is to replace the cooking and lighting methods that use charcoal and firewood with those that are "non-smoking". This can include natural gas canisters, biogas, solar, and other innovative technologies.

- If these technologies are not available it is recommended that the cooking should take place outside in the fresh air with good ventilation.

- With the creation of lower cost alternative technologies we could see small businesses that sell such things as solar stoves and lanterns make an income for the local people and reduce the prevalence of this killer disease.

- Adding some turmeric to the food and drinking neem tea for general relief from inflammation and an immune system boost.

<u>Reduction of the risk of contracting hepatitis B includes:</u>
- Taking the hepatitis B vaccine
- Using latex condoms when having sex
- Not sharing needles
- Not sharing personal care items such as toothbrushes and razors
- Avoiding tattoos and body piercings , or making sure that the artist or piercer is following good health practices.

- All pregnant women should be screened for hepatitis B and consider getting the hepatitis B vaccine. The vaccine can be given during pregnancy

- Infants who are born to women with hepatitis B should be given both hepatitis B immunoglobulin and the hepatitis B vaccine within 12 hours after birth. This can help reduce the rate of transmission of the disease to the baby.

- There are a number of drugs that can be used to treat hepatitis B, but none of them are approved for use during pregnancy.

Measures against rheumatic heart diseases

- Create prospective disease registers at sentinel sites in affected countries to measure disease burden and track progress towards the reduction of mortality by 25% by the year 20

- Ensure an adequate supply of high-quality benzathine penicillin for the primary and secondary prevention of ARF/RHD

- Improve access to reproductive health services for women with RHD and other non-communicable diseases (NCD),

- Decentralized technical expertise and technology for diagnosing and managing ARF and RHD (including Ultrasound of the heart),

- Establish national and regional centers of excellence for essential cardiac surgery for the treatment of affected patients and training of cardiovascular practitioners of the future,

- Initiate a national multi-sectoral RHD programs within NCD control programs of affected countries,

- To foster international partnerships with multinational organizations for resource mobilization, monitoring and evaluation of the program to end RHD in Africa

Measures for prevention of cancer cervix

Treatment of human papilloma virus.

Vaccines to prevent HPV infection.

- PAP smear for early cervical cancer detection.
- Practice sex in older age as it is common in young women.
- Use of condom.

- Prevent smoking.

References

1. *"South Africa - CIA - The World Factbook". https://www.cia.gov. 4 April 2007.*External link in |work= (help)

2. *"page 271" (PDF). Retrieved 15 May 2011.*

3. http://www.statssa.gov.za/publications/P0302/P03022010.pdf page 5

4. http://www.statssa.gov.za/publicationsd/P0302/P03022010.pdf page 8

5. http://www.statssa.gov.za/publications/p03093/p030932010.pdf Table 4.5

6. *"page 25-26" (PDF). Retrieved 15 May 2011.*

7. "South Africa HIV & AIDS Statistics." AVERT. Web. 3 Mar. 2012. <http://www.avert.org/south-africa-hiv-aids-statistics.htm>.

8. *"The national hiv and syphilis prevalence survey south africa 2007". The South African Department of Health. Retrieved 22 October 2008.*

9. *"Sub-Saharan Africa AIDS epidemic update. Regional Summary" (PDF). UNAIDS. Retrieved 22 October 2008.*

10. *"The Impact of HIV/AIDS on the South African Economy: A Review of Current Evidence" (PDF). TIPS. Retrieved 22 October 2008.* table on page 23

11. *"GLOBAL HEALTH INITIATIVE. Private Sector Intervention Case Example" (PDF).Daimler-Chrysler. Retrieved 22 October 2008.* page 2

12. *"page 14" (PDF). Retrieved 15 May 2011.*

13. *"Graham Mackay, CEO, SABMiller , Global Business Coalition on HIV/AIDS, Tuberculosis and Malaria". Gbcimpact.org. Retrieved 15 May 2011.*

14. *"South Africa recalls 1m ANC condoms: Scores of people given free condoms at the party's centenary celebrations have complained that they are faulty". The Guardian. 31 January 2012.*

15. *"South Africa – Country Progress Report" (PDF). Retrieved 15 May 2011.*

16. *"National HIV/AIDS and TB Unit, National Department of Health, Pretoria". Doh.gov.za. Retrieved 15 May 2011.*

17. http://www.info.gov.za/otherdocs/2007/aidsplan2007/backg round.pdf

18. Ras GJ, Simson IW, Anderson R, Prozesky OW, Hamersma T. Acquired immunodeficiency syndrome. A report of 2 South African cases. S Afr Med J 1983 Jul 23; 64(4): 140–2.

19. http://www.info.gov.za/otherdocs/2000/population/chap6.pd f

20. *"Epidemiology of HIV/AIDS in South Africa : Dr T Govender" (PDF). Retrieved 15 May2011.*

21. _"The Sarafina II Controversy". Healthlink.org.za._
    Retrieved 15 May 2011.

22. _"Zuma'S Response To Sarafina Ii". Doh.gov.za._
    Retrieved 15 May 2011.

23. _"International Conference for People Living with HIV and_
    AIDS, Cape Town, South Africa, March 6–10; Pre-
    Conference for Wo". Retrieved 15 May 2011.

24. Watkins D[1], Zuhlke L[2], Engel M[2], Daniels R[2], Francis
    V[2], Shaboodien G[2], Kango M[3], Abul-Fadl A[4], Adeoye
    A[5], Ali S[6], Al-Kebsi M[7], Bode-Thomas F[8], Bukhman
    G[9], Damasceno A[10], Goshu DY[11], Elghamrawy A[12], Gitura
    B[13], Haileamlak A[14], Hailu A[15], Hugo-Hamman C[16], Justus
    S[17], Karthikeyan G[18], Kennedy N[19],Lwabi P[20], Mamo
    Y[21], Mntla P[22], Sutton C[22], Mocumbi AO[23], Mondo
    C[24], Mtaja A[25], Musuku J[25], Mucumbitsi J[26], Murango
    L[27], Nel G[28], Ogendo S[29], Ogola E[29], Ojji D[30], Olunuga
    TO[31], Redi MM[32], Rusingiza KE[33], Sani M[34], Sheta
    S[35], Shongwe S[36], van Dam J[37], Gamra H[38], Carapetis
    J[39], Lennon D[40], Mayosi BM[41]. Seven key actions to
    eradicate rheumatic heart disease in Africa: the Addis Ababa
    communiquéCardiovasc J Afr. 2016 Jan 12;27:1-5. doi:
    10.5830/CVJA-2015-090. [Epub ahead of print]

25. The 2011 National Antenatal Sentinel HIV & syphilus
    prevalence survey in South Africa, National Department of
    Health of South Africa http://www.doh.gov.za

26. <u>b</u> *"The South African Department of Health Study, 2006".* *Avert.org. Retrieved15 May 2011.*

27. *South African National HIV Prevalence, Incidence, Behaviour and Communication Survey, 2008. Human Sciences Research Council. 2009. p. 79. ISBN 978-0-7969-2292-2. Archived from the original on 22 May 2010. Retrieved 2 December 2009.*

28. *"Epidemiological Fact Sheet on HIV and AIDS, 2008 (page 4 and 5)" (PDF). Retrieved 15 May 20***Jump up***^ "MBEKI: 13TH INTIONAL AIDS CONFERENCE". Info.gov.za. Retrieved15 May 2011.*

29. *"Controversy dogs Aids forum". BBC News. 10 July 2000. Retrieved 15 May 2011.*

30. http://www.tac.org.za/newsletter/2000/ns000908.txt

31. *Vos, Pierre De (28 May 2009). "Thabo Mbeki's strange relationship with the truth continues – Constitutionally Speaking". Constitutionallyspeaking.co.za. Retrieved15 May 2011.*

32. *"How can a virus cause a syndrome? asks Mbeki". Aegis.com. 21 September 2000. Retrieved 15 May 2011.*

33. *"South African split over Aids". BBC News. 4 April 2001. Retrieved 15 May 2011.*

34. *Blandy, Fran (16 August 2006). "'Dr Beetroot' hits back at media over Aids exhibition". Mail & Guardian Online.*

35. Garlic AIDS cure minister sidelined, 12 Sep 2006 Archived 5 January 2008 at the Wayback Machine.

36. *Lewandowsky, Mann, Bauld, Hastings, Loftus."http://www.psychologicalscience.org/index.php/publ ications/observer/2013/november-2013/the-subterranean-war-on-science.html". Observer. Association for psychological science. Retrieved 4 November 2013.*

37. Pieter Fourie "The Political Management of HIV and AIDS in South Africa: One burden too many?" Palgrave Macmillan, 2006, ISBN 0-230-00667-1

38. Fassin, Didier "When Bodies Remember: Experiences and Politics of AIDS in South Africa" University of California Press, 2007, ISBN 978-0-520-25027-7

39. *"Zapiro cartoon". Zapiro.com. 15 February 2004. Retrieved 15 May 2011.*

40. *"We don't need red hrrings". Mg.co.za. 29 September 2003. Retrieved 15 May 2011.*

41. *"Manto defends AIDS policies". Mg.co.za. 21 August 2006. Retrieved 15 May 2011.*

42. *"President heralds new era". Unaids.org. Retrieved 15 May 2011.*

43. *Duncan, C (2009). "HIV in the print media: A comparative and retrospective print media monitoring analysis".*

44. Centers for Disease Control and Prevention (CDC). HIV prevalence estimates— United States, 2006. *MMWR Morb Mortal Wkly Rep.* 2008;57(39):1073–1076.

45. Jones JL, Hanson DL, Dworkin MS, et al. Surveillance for AIDSdefining opportunistic illnesses, 1992–1997. *MMWR CDC Surveill Summ.* 1999;48(2):1–22.

46. Currier JS, Havlir DV. Complications of HIV disease and antiretroviral therapy. *Top HIV Med.* 2009;17(2):57–67.

47. Havlir DV, Currier JS. Complications of HIV disease and antiretroviral therapy. *Top HIV Med.* 2006;14(1):27–35.

48. Lesho EP, Gey DC. Managing issues related to antiretroviral therapy. *Am Fam Physician.* 2003;68(4):675–686.

49. Kaplan JE, Benson C, Holmes KH, Brooks JT, Pau A, Masur H. Guidelines for prevention and treatment of opportunistic infections in HIV-infected adults and adolescents: recommendations from CDC, the National Institutes of Health, and the HIV Medicine Association of the Infectious Diseases Society of America. *MMWR Recomm Rep.* 2009;58(RR-4):1–207.

50. González-Scarano F, Martín-García J. The neuropathogenesis of AIDS. *Nat Rev Immunol.* 2005;5(1):69–81.

51. Ellis R, Heaton R, Letendre S, et al. Higher CD4 nadir is associated with reduced rates of HIV-associated neurocognitive disorders in the CHARTER study: potential

implications for early treatment initiation. Paper presented at: 17th Conference on Retroviruses and Opportunistic Infections; February 16–19, 2010; San Francisco, Calif.

52. Bhaskaran K, Mussini C, Antinori A, et al.; CASCADE Collaboration. Changes in the incidence and predictors of human immunodeficiency virus-associated dementia in the era of highly active antiretroviral therapy. *Ann Neurol.* 2008;63(2):213–221.

53. Power C, Selnes OA, Grim JA, McArthur JC. HIV Dementia Scale: a rapid screening test. *J Acquir Immune Defic Syndr Hum Retrovirol.* 1995;8(3):273–278.

54. Davis HF, Skolasky RL Jr, Selnes OA, Burgess DM, McArthur JC. Assessing HIV-associated dementia: modified HIV dementia scale versus the Grooved Pegboard. *AIDS Read.* 2002;12(1):29–3138.

55. von Giesen HJ, Haslinger BA, Rohe S, Köller H, Arendt G. HIV Dementia Scale and psychomotor slowing—the best methods in screening for neuro-AIDS. *J Neuropsychiatry Clin Neurosci.* 2005;17(2):185–191.

56. Green DA, Masliah E, Vinters HV, Beizai P, Moore DJ, Achim CL. Brain deposition of beta-amyloid is a common pathologic feature in HIV positive patients. *AIDS.* 2005;19(4):407–411.

57. Brew BJ, Crowe SM, Landay A, Cysique LA, Guillemin G. Neurodegeneration and ageing in the HAART era. *J Neuroimmune Pharmacol.* 2009;4(2):163–174.

58. Letendre SL, Ellis RJ, Everall I, Ances B, Bharti A, McCutchan JA. Neurologic complications of HIV disease and their treatment. *Top HIV Med.* 2009;17(2):46–56.

59. Bing EG, Burnam MA, Longshore D, et al. Psychiatric disorders and drug use among human immunodeficiency virus-infected adults in the United States. *Arch Gen Psychiatry.* 2001;58(8):721–728.

60. Triant VA, Lee H, Hadigan C, Grinspoon SK. Increased acute myocardial infarction rates and cardiovascular risk factors among patients with human immunodeficiency virus disease. *J Clin Endocrinol Metab.* 2007;92(7):2506–2512.

61. Kingsley LA, Cuervo-Rojas J, Muñoz A, et al. Subclinical coronary atherosclerosis, HIV infection and antiretroviral therapy: Multicenter AIDS Cohort Study. *AIDS.* 2008;22(13):1589–1599.

62. Ross AC, Rizk N, O'Riordan MA, et al. Relationship between inflammatory markers, endothelial activation markers, and carotid intima-media thickness in HIV-infected patients receiving antiretroviral therapy. *Clin Infect Dis.* 2009;49(7):1119–1127.

63. Tesoriero JM, Gieryic SM, Carrascal A, Lavigne HE. Smoking among HIV positive New Yorkers: prevalence, frequency, and opportunities for cessation. *AIDS Behav.* 2010;14(4):824–835.

64. Behrens G, Dejam A, Schmidt H, et al. Impaired glucose tolerance, beta cell function and lipid metabolism in HIV

patients under treatment with protease inhibitors. *AIDS*. 1999;13(10):F63–F70

65. Justman JE, Benning L, Danoff A, et al. Protease inhibitor use and the incidence of diabetes mellitus in a large cohort of HIV-infected women. *J Acquir Immune Defic Syndr*. 2003;32(3):298–302.

66. Hsue PY, Hunt PW, Wu Y, et al. Association of abacavir and impaired endothelial function in treated and suppressed HIV-infected patients. *AIDS*. 2009;23(15):2021–2027.

67. Dubé MP, Stein JH, Aberg JA, et al. Guidelines for the evaluation and management of dyslipidemia in human immunodeficiency virus (HIV)-infected adults receiving antiretroviral therapy: recommendations of the HIV Medical Association of the Infectious Disease Society of America and the Adult AIDS Clinical Trials Group. *Clin Infect Dis*. 2003;37(5):613–627.

68. Eron JJ, Young B, Cooper DA, et al.; SWITCHMRK 1 and 2 investigators. Switch to a raltegravir-based regimen versus continuation of a lopinavirritonavir-based regimen in stable HIV-infected patients with suppressed viraemia (SWITCHMRK 1 and 2): two multicentre, double-blind, randomised controlled trials. *Lancet*. 2010;375(9712):396–407.

69. Pugliese A, Isnardi D, Saini A, Scarabelli T, Raddino R, Torre D. Impact of highly active antiretroviral therapy in

HIV-positive patients with cardiac involvement. *J Infect.* 2000;40(3):282–284.

70. Kaplan JE, Hanson D, Dworkin MS, et al. Epidemiology of human immunodeficiency virus-associated opportunistic infections in the United States in the era of highly active antiretroviral therapy. *Clin Infect Dis.* 2000;30(suppl 1):S5–S14.

71. Masur H, Shelhamer J. Empiric outpatient management of HIV-related pneumonia: economical or unwise? *Ann Intern Med.* 1996;124(4):451–453.

72. Wilkin A, Feinberg J. *Pneumocystis carinii* pneumonia: a clinical review *Am Fam Physician.* 1999;60(6):1699–1708.

73. Sitbon O, Lascoux-Combe C, Delfraissy JF, et al. Prevalence of HIV-related pulmonary arterial hypertension in the current antiretroviral therapy era. *Am J Respir Crit Care Med.* 2008;177(1):108–113.

74. Spano JP, Massiani MA, Bentata M, et al. Lung cancer in patients with HIV infection and review of the literature. *Med Oncol.* 2004;21(2):109–115.

75. Diaz PT, King ER, Wewers MD, et al. HIV infection increases susceptibility to smoking-induced emphysema. *Chest.* 2000;117(5 suppl 1):285S.

76. Kirk GD, Merlo C, O'Driscoll P, et al. HIV infection is associated with an increased risk for lung cancer, independent of smoking. *Clin Infect Dis.* 2007;45(1):103–110.

77. Wilcox CM, Saag MS. Gastrointestinal complications of HIV infection: changing priorities in the HAART era. *Gut.* 2008;57

78. Cameron JE, Hagensee ME. Oral HPV complications in HIV-infected patients. *Curr HIV/AIDS Rep.* 2008;5(3):126–131

79. Gillison ML. Oropharyngeal cancer: a potential consequence of concomitant HPV and HIV infection. *Curr Opin Oncol.* 2009;21(5):439–444.

80. Knox TA, Spiegelman D, Skinner SC, Gorbach S. Diarrhea and abnormalities of gastrointestinal function in a cohort of men and women with HIV infection. *Am J Gastroenterol.* 2000;95(12):3482–3489.

81. Zeitz M, Ullrich R, Schneider T, Kewenig S, Hohloch K, Riecken EO. HIV/SIV enteropathy. *Ann N Y Acad Sci.* 1998;859139–148.

82. Landy J, Gazzard B, Harbord M. Inflammatory bowel disease in HIV seropositive individuals: analysis of a large cohort. Paper presented at: Digestive Disease Week; May 17–22, 2008; San Diego, Calif

83. . Zar FA, El-Bayoumi E, Yungbluth MM. Histologic proof of acalculous cholecystitis due to*Cyclospora cayetanensis*. *Clin Infect Dis.* 2001;33(12):E140–E141

84. Palella FJ Jr, Baker RK, Moorman AC, et al.; HIV Outpatient Study Investigators. Mortality in the highly active antiretroviral therapy era: changing causes of death and

disease in the HIV outpatient study. *J Acquir Immune Defic Syndr*. 2006;43(1):27–34.

85. Aberg JA, Kaplan JE, Libman H, et al. Primary care guidelines for the management of persons infected with human immunodeficiency virus: 2009 update by the HIV Medicine Association of the Infectious Diseases Society of America. *Clin Infect Dis*. 2009;49(5):651–681.

86. Centers for Disease Control and Prevention (CDC) Measles. In: Atkinson W, Wolfe S, Hamborsky J, editors.Epidemiology and Prevention of Vaccine-Preventable Diseases. 12th ed. Public Health Foundation; Washington, DC: 2011. pp. 173–192

87. Center for Disease Control and Prevention (CDC) Mumps. In: Atkinson W, Wolfe S, Hamborsky J, editors.Epidemiology and Prevention of Vaccine-Preventable Diseases. 12th ed. Public Health Foundation; Washington, DC: 2011. pp. 205–214.

88. Center for Disease Control and Prevention (CDC) Rubella. In: Atkinson W, Wolfe S, Hamborsky J, editors.Epidemiology and Prevention of Vaccine-Preventable Diseases. 12th ed. Public Health Foundation; Washington, DC: 2011. pp. 275–290.

89. Watson JC, Hadler SC, Dykewicz CA, et al. Measles, mumps, and rubella--vaccine use and strategies for elimination of measles, rubella, and congenital rubella syndrome and control of mumps: recommendations of the

Advisory Committee on Immunization Practices (ACIP). MMWR Recomm Rep. 1998;47:1–57. [PubMed]

90. Gershon AA. Chickenpox, measles, and mumps. In: Remington JS, Klein JO, Wilson CB, et al., editors.Infectious Diseases of the Fetus and Newborn Infant. 7th ed. Elsevier; Philadelphia: 2011. pp. 661–705.

91. Plotkin SA, Reef SE, Cooper LZ, et al. Rubella. In: Remington JS, Klein JO, Wilson CB, et al., editors.Infectious Diseases of the Fetus and Newborn Infant. 7th ed. Elsevier; Philadelphia: 2011. pp. 861–898.

92. American Academy of Pediatrics (AAP) Committee on Fetus and Newborn and the American College of Obstetrics and Gynecology (ACOG) Committee on Obstetric Practice . Guide to Perinatal Care. 6th ed. Washington, DC: 2007. Perinatal Infections. pp. 303–348.

93. Ornoy A, Tenenbaum A. Pregnancy outcome following infections by coxsackie, echo, measles, mumps, hepatitis, polio and encephalitis viruses. Reprod Toxicol. 2006;21:446–457. [PubMed]

94. Eberhart-Phillips JE, Frederick PD, Baron RC, et al. Measles in pregnancy: a descriptive study of 58 cases.Obstet Gynecol. 1993;82:797–801. [PubMed]

95. Centers for Disease Control and Prevention (CDC) Update: Measles --- United States, January--July 2008.MMWR Morb Mortal Wkly Rep. 2008;57:893–896. [PubMed]

96. Centers for Disease Control and Prevention (CDC) Mumps Outbreak --- New York, New Jersey, Quebec, 2009. MMWR Morb Mortal Wkly Rep. 2009;58:1270–1274. [PubMed]

97. Reef SE, Strebel P, Dabbagh A, et al. Progress toward control of rubella and prevention of congenital rubella syndrome--worldwide, 2009. J Infect Dis. 2011;204:S24–27. [PubMed]

98. Valente P, Sever JL. In utero diagnosis of congenital infections by direct fetal sampling. Isr J Med Sci.1994;30:414–420. [PubMed

99. Merck & Co., Inc. [November 20, 2011];M-M-R II® (measles, mumps, and rubella vaccine live) [Merck web site] http://www.merck.com/product/usa/pi_circulars/m/mmr_ii/mmr_ii_pi.pdf

100.   Feinberg M. [November 11, 2011];Monovalent vaccines no longer available for measles, mumps, rubella [Merck vaccines web site] 2009 Oct 21; https://www.merckvaccines.com/monovalentMessage_1 02109.pdf.

101.   National Center for Immunization and Respiratory Diseases General recommendations on immunization --- recommendations of the Advisory Committee on Immunization Practices (ACIP). MMWR Recomm Rep.2011;60:1–64. [PubMed]

102.   Centers for Disease Control and Prevention (CDC) Measles Prevention. MMWR Morb Mortal Wkly Rep.1989;38:1–18.

103.   Center for Disease Control and Prevention (CDC) Update: vaccine side effects, adverse reactions, contraindications, and precautions recommendations of the Advisory Committee on Immunization Practices (ACIP). MMWR Morb Mortal Wkly Rep. 1996;45:1–35. [PubMed]

104.   LeBaron CW, Forghani B, Matter L, et al. Persistence of rubella antibodies after 2 doses of measles-mumps-rubella vaccine. J Infect Dis. 2009;200:888–899. [PubMed]

105.   Gall SA, Poland GA. A maternal immunization program (MIP): Developing a schedule and platform for routine immunization during pregnancy. Vaccine. 2011;29:9411–9413. [PubMed]

106.   Zöllner J[1], Curry R, Johnson M The contribution of heart disease to maternal mortality. Curr Opin Obstet Gynecol. 2013 Apr; 25 (2): 91-7. Do: 10.1097/GCO.0b013e32835e0f11.

www.ingramcontent.com/pod-product-compliance
Lightning Source LLC
Chambersburg PA
CBHW060406190526
45169CB00002B/781